WELCOME

CW00522233

This Food Diary Has Been Designed To Be Compatible With Your You will soon find it a super aid in your quest to lose weight and this Food Diary will become part of your day, and the helpful organised pages you on track, focused and in control.

FOOD DIARY PAGE

This Food Diary has been designed to match your plan and any food variations.
Optional: Simply use the blank column headers at the top of each page to match your current plan choice. **For example:** Free Food, Healthy, Speed, Proteins, Carbs, Shakes, porridge, soups and so on. You can also use the blank header for * Fasting Day if you follow the fast 800 or 5:2 diet plan.

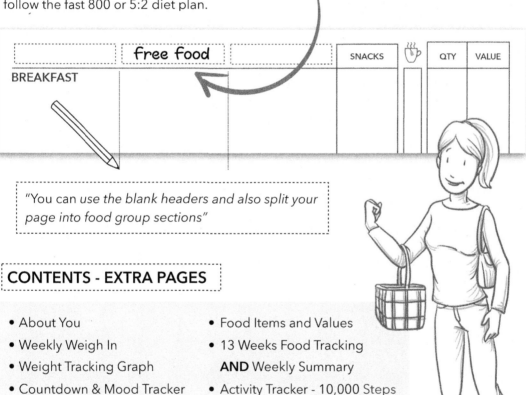

"You can *use the blank headers and also split your page into food group sections*"

CONTENTS - EXTRA PAGES

- About You
- Weekly Weigh In
- Weight Tracking Graph
- Countdown & Mood Tracker
- My Happy List
- Keep Busy - Get it done
- Keep Active

- Food Items and Values
- 13 Weeks Food Tracking **AND** Weekly Summary
- Activity Tracker - 10,000 Steps
- Exercise Information
- Exercise Log Pages
- Sleep Tracker

ABOUT ME

⭐ **ABOUT ME:** *Write down the things I like, what makes me, me?*

⭐ **MY GOALS:** *What are my goals... What motivates me?*

⭐ **WHY:** *Write down why I want to make changes in my life.*

⭐ **RELAX:** *What can I do to relax and unwind?*

⭐ **PLAN & TREAT:** *Have something to look forward to - My plans are?*

⭐ **HELP:** *Who can I talk to, who is going to support and help me?*

FOCUS: *Statement to myself to keep me motivated and focused!*

WEEKLY WEIGHT IN - Weeks 1 - 8

Happy With This Weeks Results? "Tick Your Scales"		*Weight:*
WEEK 1 - Date:		
"Did You Have A Good Result ?"		
WEEK 2 - Date:		
"Did You Have A Good Result ?"		
WEEK 3 - Date:		
"Did You Have A Good Result ?"		
WEEK 4 - Date:		
"Did You Have A Good Result ?"		
WEEK 5 - Date:		
"Did You Have A Good Result ?"		
WEEK 6 - Date:		
"Did You Have A Good Result ?"		
WEEK 7 - Date:		
"Did You Have A Good Result ?"		
WEEK 8 - Date:		
"Did You Have A Good Result ?"		

WEEKLY WEIGHT IN - Weeks 9 - 12

Happy With This Weeks Results? "Tick Your Scales"	Weight:
WEEK 9 - Date:	
"Did You Have A Good Result ?"	
WEEK 10 - Date:	
"Did You Have A Good Result ?"	
WEEK 11 - Date:	
"Did You Have A Good Result ?"	
WEEK 12 - Date:	
"Did You Have A Good Result ?"	

NOTES

MEASUREMENTS AND WEIGHT TRACKING GRAPH

Enter your "**Stone**" Weight only in **Box A** - then mark on the graph your "**Pound**" Weight!

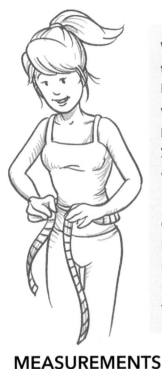

When measuring yourself with the measuring tape, the tape should fit snugly against the surface of your skin. It should not press into the skin at any point. When wrapped around you, the measuring tape should be parallel with the floor, and not askew. When measuring your bust/chest, you'll get the best results if both arms are at your side. You may need assistance for this!

Getting the same result, does not mean you haven't lost any weight. Remember your measurements are only guide lines.
Measure yourself **TODAY**, (Week 1), then weeks 3, 5, 7, 9 & 12

Box A

MEASUREMENTS

WEEKS

Neck	Arm **L**	Arm **R**	Bust	Waist	Thigh **L**	Thigh **R**	Calf **L**	Calf **R**	
									1
									3
									5
									7
									9
									12

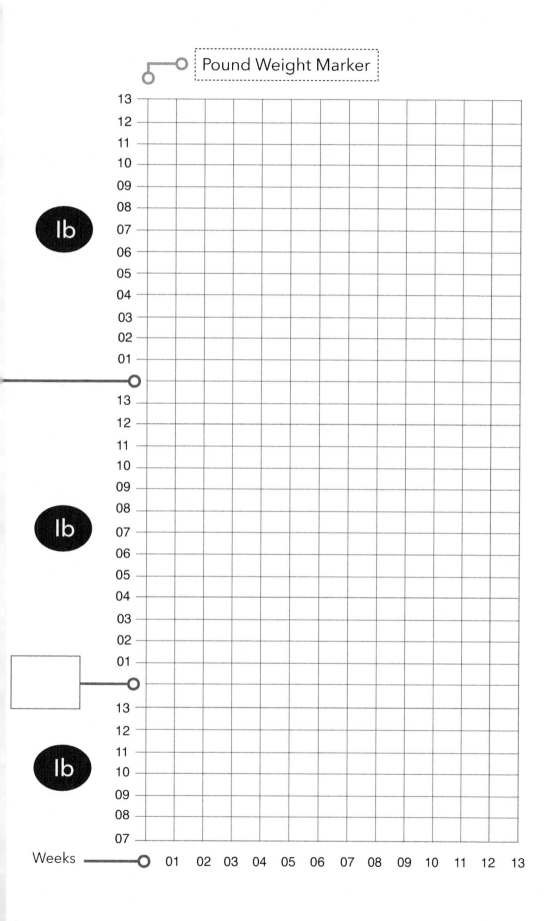

Pound Weight Marker

lb

lb

lb

Weeks ── 01 02 03 04 05 06 07 08 09 10 11 12 13

COUNTDOWN & MOOD TRACKER

12 Weeks Line a Smile or Don't!

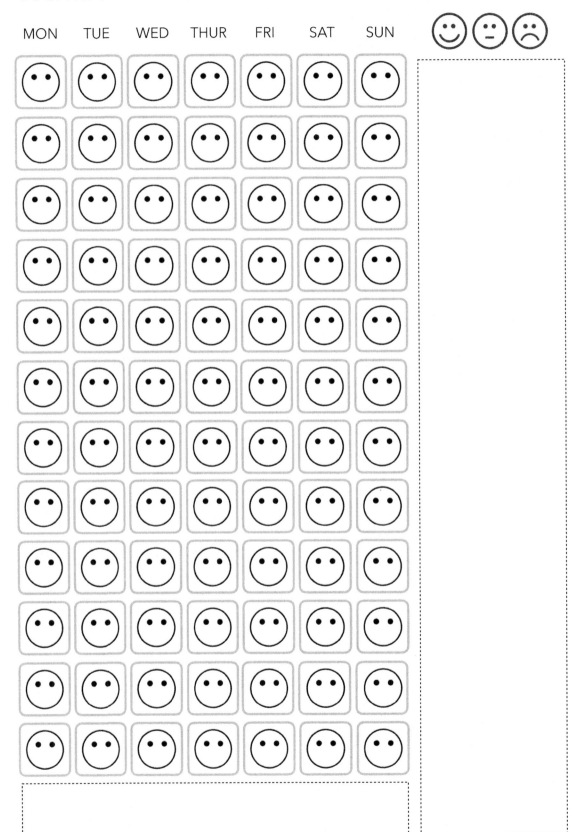

A beautiful list of things that make me feel happy…!

GET IT DONE...! Active Body & Mind - Jobs that will keep me busy!

- [ ]
- [ ]
- [ ]
- [ ]
- [ ]
- [ ]
- [ ]
- [ ]
- [ ]
- [ ]
- [ ]
- [ ]
- [ ]

NOTES

Activities that will help keep me busy!

NOTES

TICKS AND BEVERAGES

Your beverages are just as important as your meals. Lots of people who are on a diet forget that beverages contain Calories.   Some people drink more beverages than others. Sometimes this may be a work environment factor or simply drinking becomes a habit rather than a need.

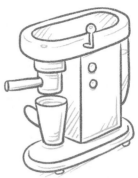

 ## "Counting ticks is like counting Calories"

If we all took in fluids for our needs only, we would only drink water. This would be a good thing, but we don't simply drink to nourish and hydrate our bodies anymore, we drink for flavour, enjoyment and socialising.

Beverages taste nice and supply us with a little boost or kick we are looking for. The most common beverages are, you guessed it, tea, coffee and hot chocolate.

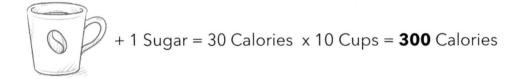

+ 1 Sugar = 30 Calories x 10 Cups = **300** Calories

The reason you need to place a tick on your Diary page each time you have a beverage, is so you can see at a glance how many beverages you are having!

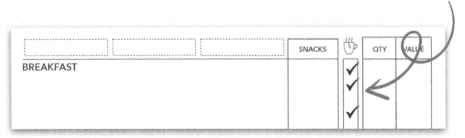

			SNACKS	☕	QTY	VALUE
BREAKFAST				✓		
				✓		
				✓		

You may be shocked at the amount you do have. Reducing your beverages alone may be all the difference you're looking for to lose weight.

Simply looking at the number of ticks on your page may give you a true picture to whether you are just having too many, or too many in one particular part of the day. You may be able to say to yourself - NO more coffees in the morning, or I will at least reduce this by half!

BEVERAGES AND REDUCING SUGAR EASILY

I suggest for the first week of your diet you stick with you normal number of beverages. Then look back at the end of the week and find the pattern to see how you can realistically reduce the number. You don't want to lose too much of something you love, so start by setting a lower goal target and work it from there.

You will be amazed at how reducing your beverages has a marked impact on your weight loss, especially if you have sugar in your tea or coffee.

If you do have sugar in your tea or coffee and you are counting calories, use a measuring spoon instead of a teaspoon. A tea spoon of sugar can vary so much that over time your calorie count can be out by a lot!

Your spoonful may be bigger than mine!

A spoonful of sugar (1tsp 4.2g) is 16 calories. But is your spoonful 16 calories or more? There could be a 5 to 15 calorie difference if your spoonful is heaped. Times this by ten cups and your calorie count is out by as much as 150 calories! (1050 calories per week).

16 Calories…   *28 Calories…*

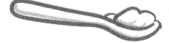 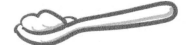

It all sounds a little "Picky" but it really does make the difference. When reducing your sugar, don't simply cut it out. Reduce it slowly over a few weeks, using level measuring spoons. This way your taste buds will get used to the small reductions and in a few weeks you can be using the smallest of measuring spoons and your beverage will still taste as sweet. Your beverage will taste just as nice, but you will be getting a fraction of the calories. You may even decide you prefer your drinks with no sugar at all!

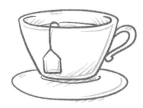

FOOD VALUE REMINDERS

Write down your most used food items and the values.

ITEM	VALUE	ITEM	VALUE

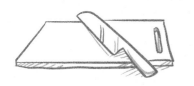   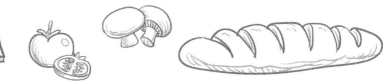

ITEM	VALUE	ITEM	VALUE

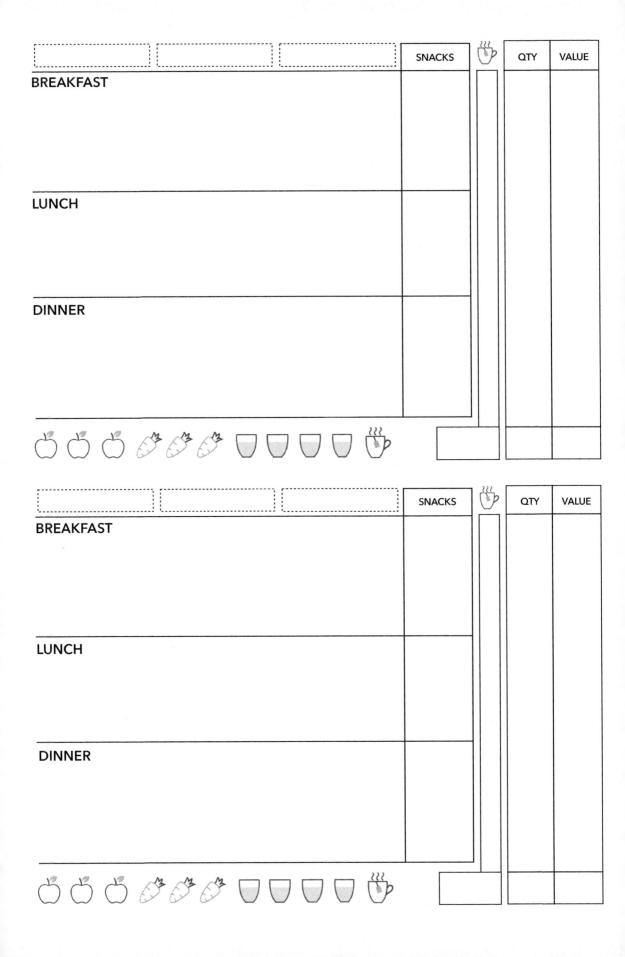

			SNACKS		QTY	VALUE

BREAKFAST

LUNCH

DINNER

			SNACKS		QTY	VALUE

BREAKFAST

LUNCH

DINNER

			SNACKS	☕	QTY	VALUE
BREAKFAST						
LUNCH						
DINNER						

🍎 🍎 🍎 🥕 🥕 🥕 🥛 🥛 🥛 🥛 ☕

			SNACKS	☕	QTY	VALUE
BREAKFAST						
LUNCH						
DINNER						

🍎 🍎 🍎 🥕 🥕 🥕 🥛 🥛 🥛 🥛 ☕

			SNACKS		QTY	VALUE

BREAKFAST

LUNCH

DINNER

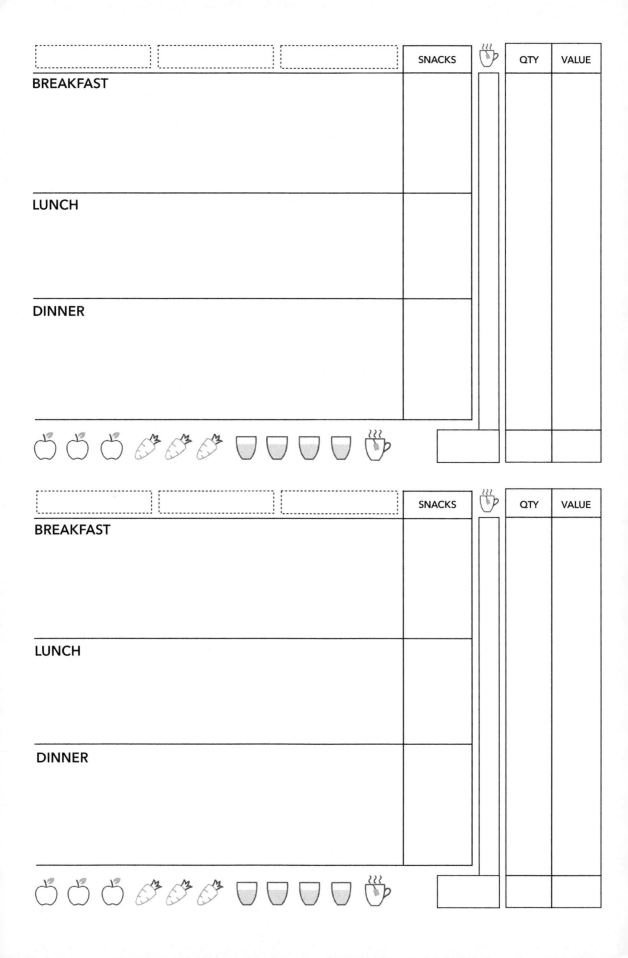

			SNACKS		QTY	VALUE

BREAKFAST

LUNCH

DINNER

			SNACKS	☕	QTY	VALUE
BREAKFAST						
LUNCH						
DINNER						

🍎 🍎 🍎 🥕 🥕 🥕 🥤 🥤 🥤 🥤 ☕

WEEK 1 - SEVEN DAY SUMMARY

	VALUE TOTALS	BEVERAGE TOTALS

Fruit - Veg - Water

- MONDAY • ___ ___ ___   • ___   • ___
- TUESDAY • ___ ___ ___   • ___   • ___
- WEDNESDAY • ___ ___ ___   • ___   • ___
- THURSDAY • ___ ___ ___   • ___   • ___
- FRIDAY • ___ ___ ___   • ___   • ___
- SATURDAY • ___ ___ ___   • ___   • ___
- SUNDAY • ___ ___ ___   • ___   • ___

GRAND TOTALS ➡ ___ ___ ___   ➡ ___   ➡ ___

			SNACKS		QTY	VALUE

BREAKFAST

LUNCH

DINNER

			SNACKS		QTY	VALUE

BREAKFAST

LUNCH

DINNER

			SNACKS	☕	QTY	VALUE
BREAKFAST						
LUNCH						
DINNER						

🍎 🍎 🍎 🥕 🥕 🥕 ☕ ☕ ☕ ☕ ☕

			SNACKS	☕	QTY	VALUE
BREAKFAST						
LUNCH						
DINNER						

🍎 🍎 🍎 🥕 🥕 🥕 ☕ ☕ ☕ ☕ ☕

			SNACKS	☕	QTY	VALUE

BREAKFAST

LUNCH

DINNER

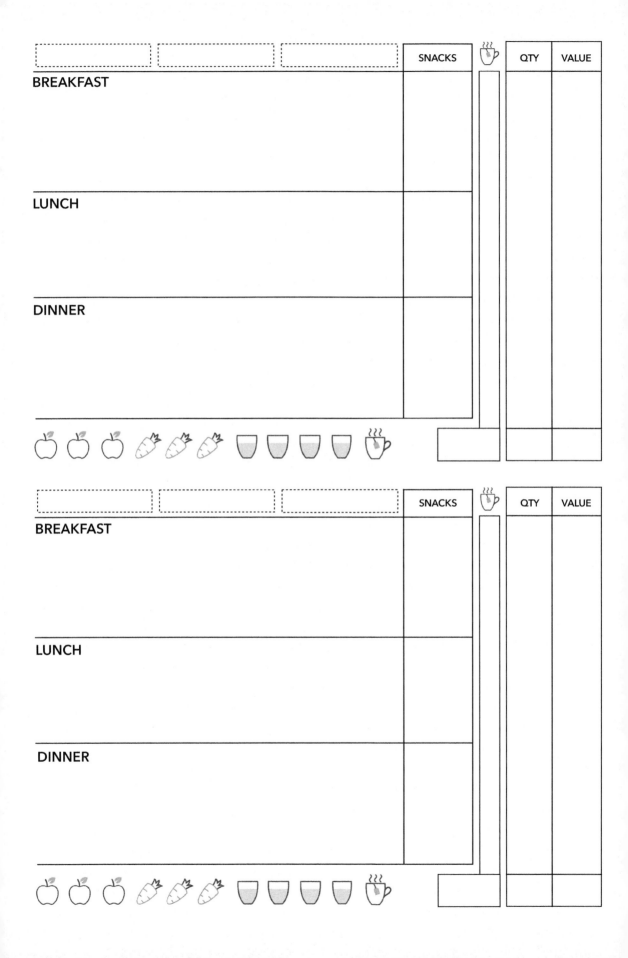

			SNACKS	☕	QTY	VALUE

BREAKFAST

LUNCH

DINNER

			SNACKS	☕	QTY	VALUE
BREAKFAST						
LUNCH						
DINNER						

🍎 🍎 🍎 🥕 🥕 🥕 ☕ ☕ ☕ ☕ ☕

WEEK 2 - SEVEN DAY SUMMARY

	VALUE TOTALS	BEVERAGE TOTALS

Fruit - Veg - Water

- MONDAY • ___ ___ ___   • ___   • ___
- TUESDAY • ___ ___ ___   • ___   • ___
- WEDNESDAY • ___ ___ ___   • ___   • ___
- THURSDAY • ___ ___ ___   • ___   • ___
- FRIDAY • ___ ___ ___   • ___   • ___
- SATURDAY • ___ ___ ___   • ___   • ___
- SUNDAY • ___ ___ ___   • ___   • ___

GRAND TOTALS ➡ ___ ___ ___   ➡ ___   ➡ ___

			SNACKS	☕	QTY	VALUE
BREAKFAST						
LUNCH						
DINNER						

🍎 🍎 🍎 🥕 🥕 🥕 🥤 🥤 🥤 🥤 ☕

			SNACKS	☕	QTY	VALUE
BREAKFAST						
LUNCH						
DINNER						

🍎 🍎 🍎 🥕 🥕 🥕 🥤 🥤 🥤 🥤 ☕

			SNACKS		QTY	VALUE

BREAKFAST

LUNCH

DINNER

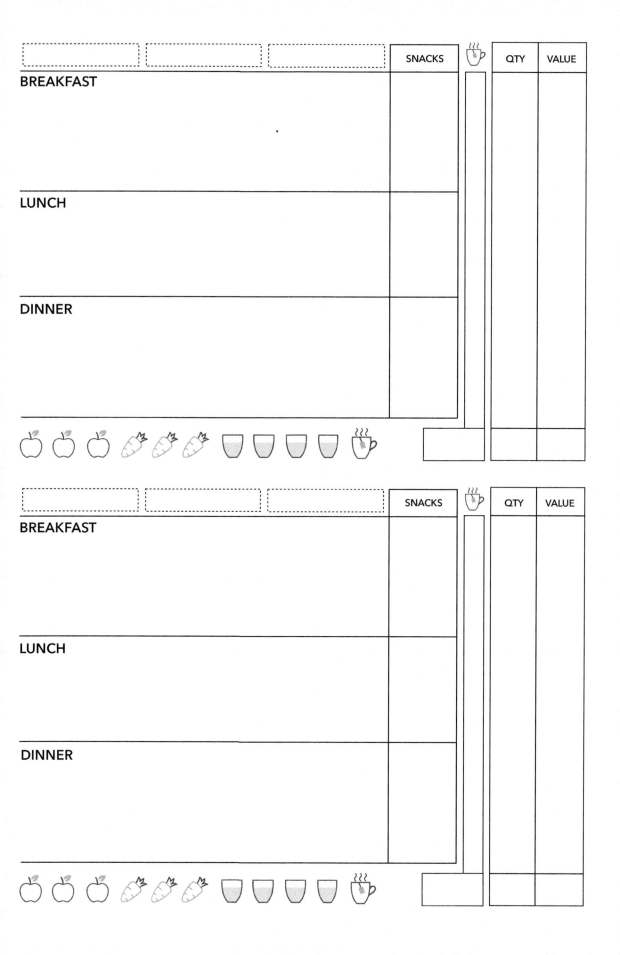

			SNACKS		QTY	VALUE

BREAKFAST

LUNCH

DINNER

			SNACKS		QTY	VALUE

BREAKFAST

LUNCH

DINNER

			SNACKS		QTY	VALUE

BREAKFAST

LUNCH

DINNER

			SNACKS	☕	QTY	VALUE
BREAKFAST						
LUNCH						
DINNER						

🍎 🍎 🍎 🥕 🥕 🥕 ☕ ☕ ☕ ☕ ☕

WEEK 3 - SEVEN DAY SUMMARY

	VALUE TOTALS	BEVERAGE TOTALS

Fruit - Veg - Water

- MONDAY ● ___ ___ ___   ● ___   ● ___
- TUESDAY ● ___ ___ ___   ● ___   ● ___
- WEDNESDAY ● ___ ___ ___   ● ___   ● ___
- THURSDAY ● ___ ___ ___   ● ___   ● ___
- FRIDAY ● ___ ___ ___   ● ___   ● ___
- SATURDAY ● ___ ___ ___   ● ___   ● ___
- SUNDAY ● ___ ___ ___   ● ___   ● ___

GRAND TOTALS ➡ ___ ___ ___   ➡ ___   ➡ ___

			SNACKS	☕	QTY	VALUE
BREAKFAST						
LUNCH						
DINNER						

🍎 🍎 🍎 🥕 🥕 🥕 🥤 🥤 🥤 🥤 ☕

			SNACKS	☕	QTY	VALUE
BREAKFAST						
LUNCH						
DINNER						

🍎 🍎 🍎 🥕 🥕 🥕 🥤 🥤 🥤 🥤 ☕

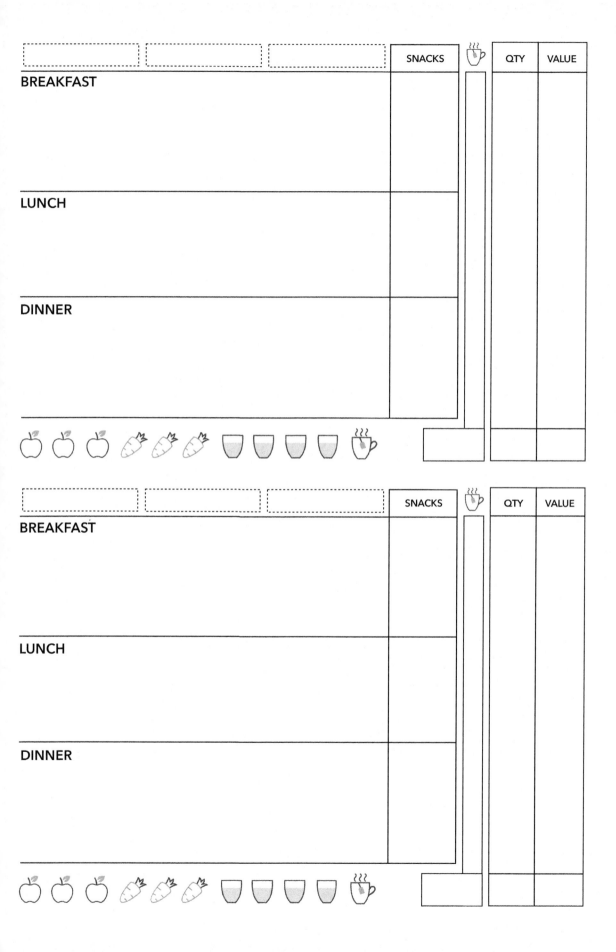

			SNACKS		QTY	VALUE
BREAKFAST						
LUNCH						
DINNER						

			SNACKS		QTY	VALUE
BREAKFAST						
LUNCH						
DINNER						

			SNACKS	☕	QTY	VALUE
BREAKFAST						
LUNCH						
DINNER						

🍎 🍎 🍎 🥕 🥕 🥕 🥤 🥤 🥤 🥤 ☕

			SNACKS	☕	QTY	VALUE
BREAKFAST						
LUNCH						
DINNER						

🍎 🍎 🍎 🥕 🥕 🥕 🥤 🥤 🥤 🥤 ☕

			SNACKS	☕	QTY	VALUE
BREAKFAST						
LUNCH						
DINNER						

🍎 🍎 🍎 🥕 🥕 🥕 🥛 🥛 🥛 🥛 ☕

WEEK 4 - SEVEN DAY SUMMARY

	VALUE TOTALS	BEVERAGE TOTALS

Fruit - Veg - Water

- MONDAY • ___ ___ ___   • ___   • ___
- TUESDAY • ___ ___ ___   • ___   • ___
- WEDNESDAY • ___ ___ ___   • ___   • ___
- THURSDAY • ___ ___ ___   • ___   • ___
- FRIDAY • ___ ___ ___   • ___   • ___
- SATURDAY • ___ ___ ___   • ___   • ___
- SUNDAY • ___ ___ ___   • ___   • ___

GRAND TOTALS ➡ ___ ___ ___   ➡ ___   ➡ ___

			SNACKS		QTY	VALUE

BREAKFAST

LUNCH

DINNER

			SNACKS		QTY	VALUE

BREAKFAST

LUNCH

DINNER

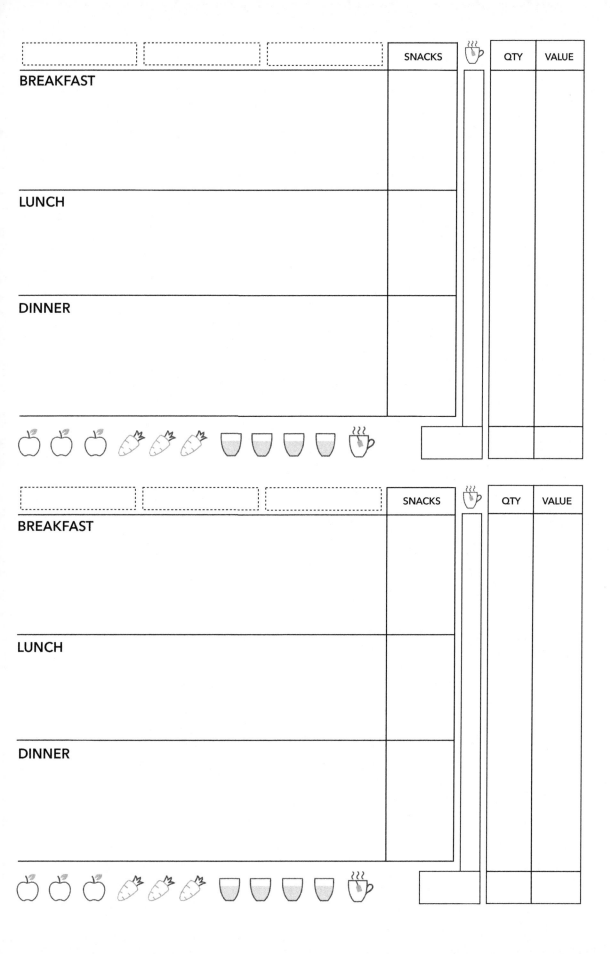

			SNACKS	☕	QTY	VALUE
BREAKFAST						
LUNCH						
DINNER						

			SNACKS	☕	QTY	VALUE
BREAKFAST						
LUNCH						
DINNER						

			SNACKS	☕	QTY	VALUE

BREAKFAST

LUNCH

DINNER

			SNACKS	☕	QTY	VALUE

BREAKFAST

LUNCH

DINNER

			SNACKS	☕	QTY	VALUE
BREAKFAST						
LUNCH						
DINNER						

🍎 🍎 🍎 🥕 🥕 🥕 🥛 🥛 🥛 🥛 ☕

WEEK 5 - SEVEN DAY SUMMARY

	Fruit - Veg - Water	VALUE TOTALS	BEVERAGE TOTALS
• MONDAY	• ___ ___ ___	• ___	• ___
• TUESDAY	• ___ ___ ___	• ___	• ___
• WEDNESDAY	• ___ ___ ___	• ___	• ___
• THURSDAY	• ___ ___ ___	• ___	• ___
• FRIDAY	• ___ ___ ___	• ___	• ___
• SATURDAY	• ___ ___ ___	• ___	• ___
• SUNDAY	• ___ ___ ___	• ___	• ___

GRAND TOTALS ➤ ___ ___ ➤ ___ ➤ ___

			SNACKS	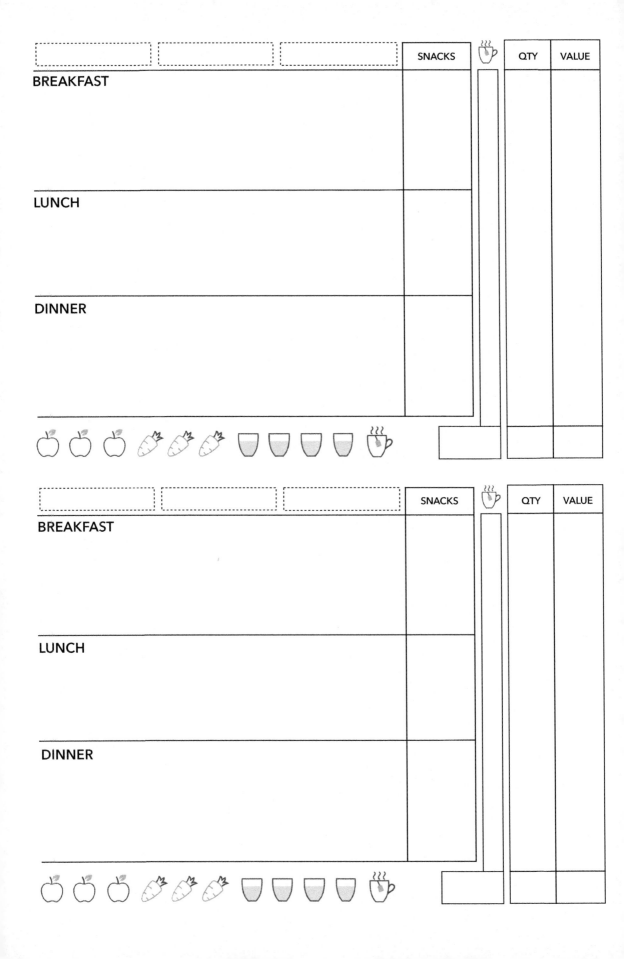	QTY	VALUE

BREAKFAST

LUNCH

DINNER

			SNACKS		QTY	VALUE

BREAKFAST

LUNCH

DINNER

			SNACKS	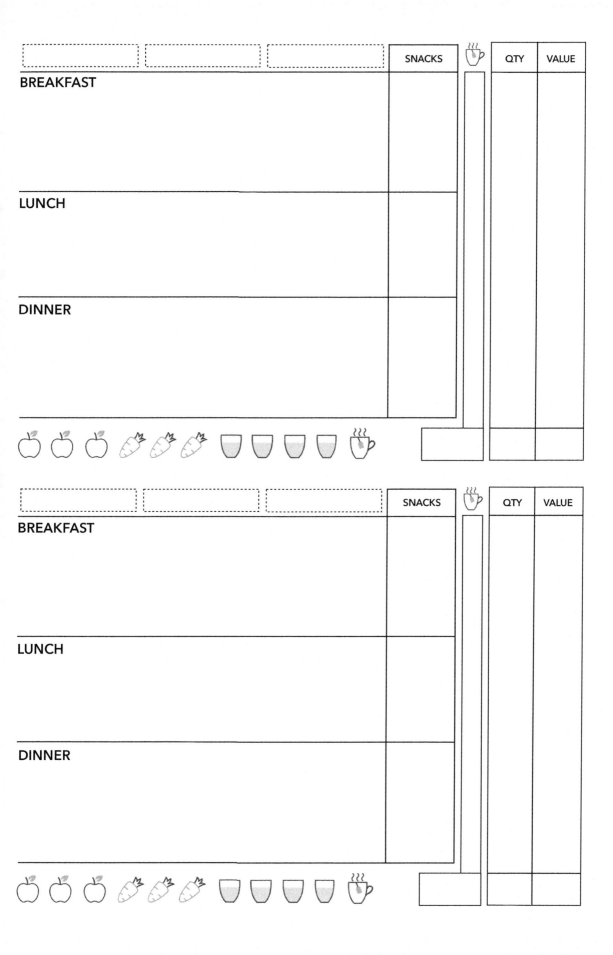	QTY	VALUE

BREAKFAST

LUNCH

DINNER

			SNACKS		QTY	VALUE

BREAKFAST

LUNCH

DINNER

			SNACKS	☕	QTY	VALUE
BREAKFAST						
LUNCH						
DINNER						

🍎 🍎 🍎 🥕 🥕 🥕 🥛 🥛 🥛 🥛 ☕

			SNACKS	☕	QTY	VALUE
BREAKFAST						
LUNCH						
DINNER						

🍎 🍎 🍎 🥕 🥕 🥕 🥛 🥛 🥛 🥛 ☕

			SNACKS	☕	QTY	VALUE
BREAKFAST						
LUNCH						
DINNER						

🍎 🍎 🍎 🥕 🥕 🥕 🥛 🥛 🥛 🥛 ☕

WEEK 6 - SEVEN DAY SUMMARY

	VALUE TOTALS	BEVERAGE TOTALS

Fruit - Veg - Water

- MONDAY ● ____ ____ ____   ● ____   ● ____
- TUESDAY ● ____ ____ ____   ● ____   ● ____
- WEDNESDAY ● ____ ____ ____   ● ____   ● ____
- THURSDAY ● ____ ____ ____   ● ____   ● ____
- FRIDAY ● ____ ____ ____   ● ____   ● ____
- SATURDAY ● ____ ____ ____   ● ____   ● ____
- SUNDAY ● ____ ____ ____   ● ____   ● ____

GRAND TOTALS ➤ ____ ____ ____   ➤ ____   ➤ ____

			SNACKS	☕	QTY	VALUE
BREAKFAST						
LUNCH						
DINNER						

🍎 🍎 🍎 🥕 🥕 🥕 🥤 🥤 🥤 🥤 ☕

			SNACKS	☕	QTY	VALUE
BREAKFAST						
LUNCH						
DINNER						

🍎 🍎 🍎 🥕 🥕 🥕 🥤 🥤 🥤 🥤 ☕

			SNACKS		QTY	VALUE
BREAKFAST						
LUNCH						
DINNER						

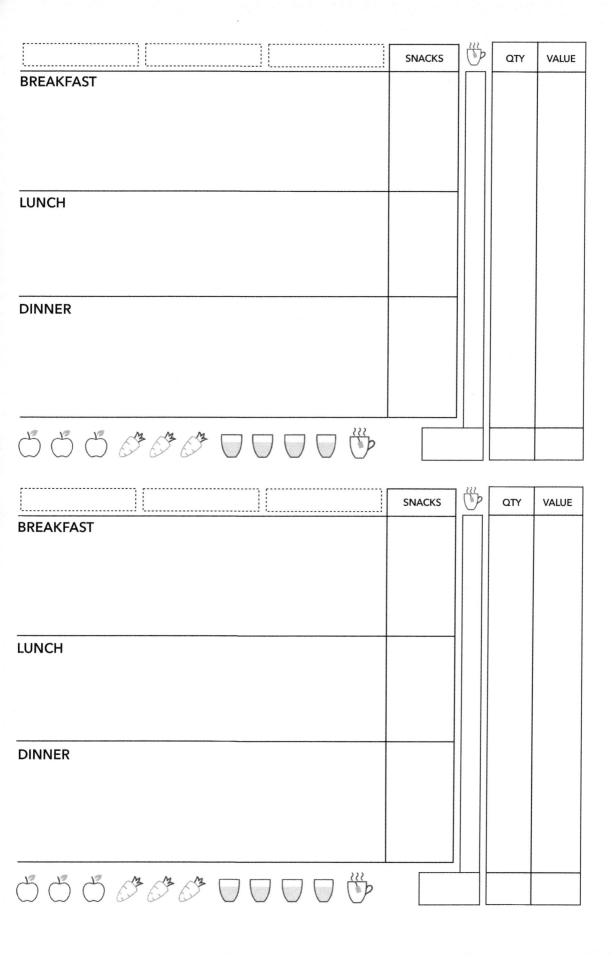

			SNACKS		QTY	VALUE
BREAKFAST						
LUNCH						
DINNER						

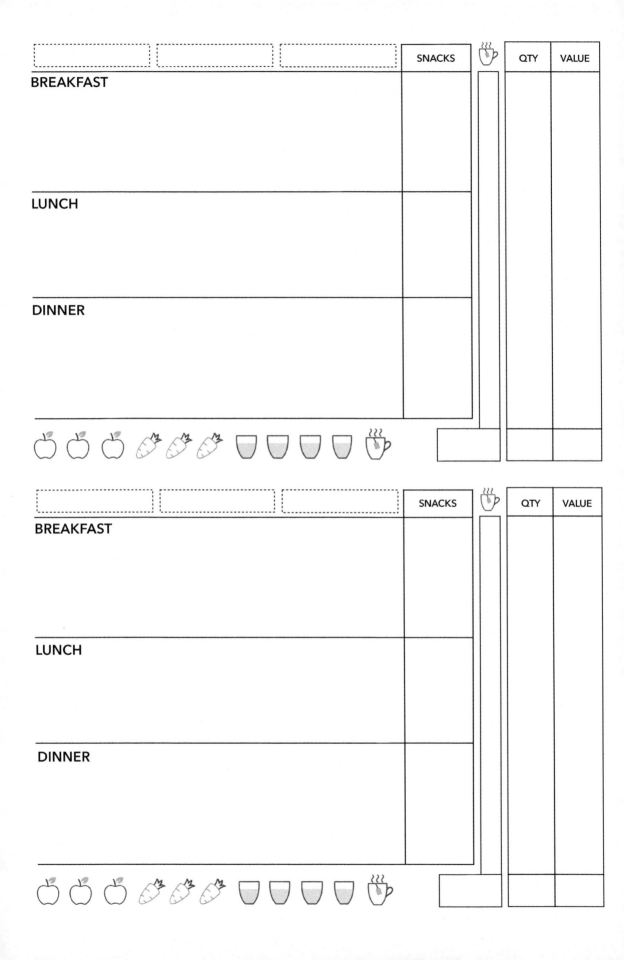

			SNACKS		QTY	VALUE

BREAKFAST

LUNCH

DINNER

			SNACKS		QTY	VALUE

BREAKFAST

LUNCH

DINNER

			SNACKS	☕	QTY	VALUE
BREAKFAST						
LUNCH						
DINNER						

🍎 🍎 🍎 🥕 🥕 🥕 🥛 🥛 🥛 🥛 ☕

WEEK 7 - SEVEN DAY SUMMARY

	VALUE TOTALS	BEVERAGE TOTALS

Fruit - Veg - Water

- MONDAY
- TUESDAY
- WEDNESDAY
- THURSDAY
- FRIDAY
- SATURDAY
- SUNDAY

GRAND TOTALS ▶

			SNACKS	☕	QTY	VALUE
BREAKFAST						
LUNCH						
DINNER						

🍎 🍎 🍎 🥕 🥕 🥕 🥤 🥤 🥤 🥤 ☕

			SNACKS	☕	QTY	VALUE
BREAKFAST						
LUNCH						
DINNER						

🍎 🍎 🍎 🥕 🥕 🥕 🥤 🥤 🥤 🥤 ☕

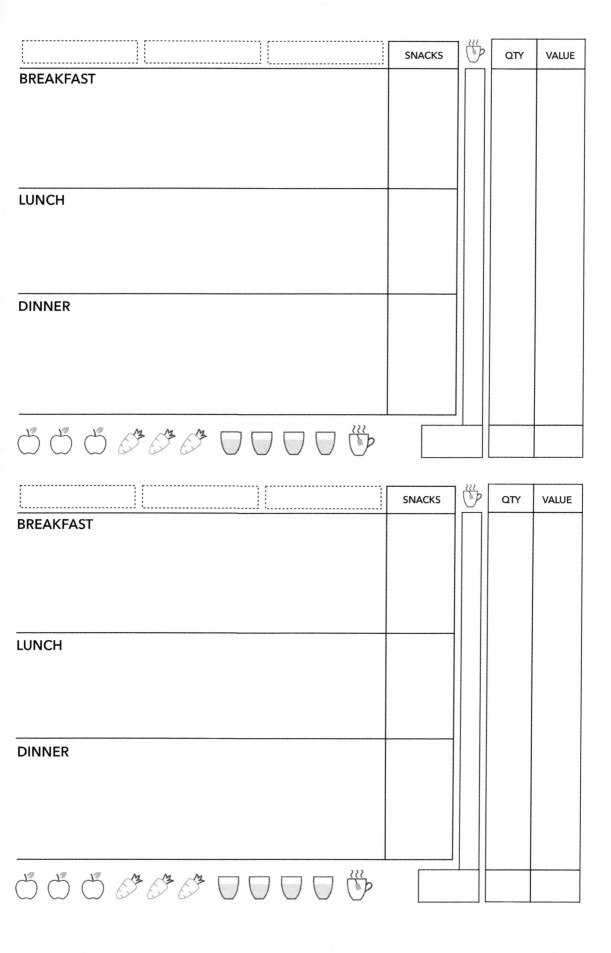

			SNACKS		QTY	VALUE
BREAKFAST						
LUNCH						
DINNER						

			SNACKS		QTY	VALUE
BREAKFAST						
LUNCH						
DINNER						

			SNACKS	☕	QTY	VALUE
BREAKFAST						
LUNCH						
DINNER						

🍎 🍎 🍎 🥕 🥕 🥕 🥤 🥤 🥤 🥤 ☕

			SNACKS	☕	QTY	VALUE
BREAKFAST						
LUNCH						
DINNER						

🍎 🍎 🍎 🥕 🥕 🥕 🥤 🥤 🥤 🥤 ☕

			SNACKS	☕	QTY	VALUE
BREAKFAST						
LUNCH						
DINNER						

🍎 🍎 🍎 🥕 🥕 🥕 🥤 🥤 🥤 🥤 ☕

WEEK 8 - SEVEN DAY SUMMARY

		VALUE TOTALS	BEVERAGE TOTALS

Fruit - Veg - Water

- MONDAY
- TUESDAY
- WEDNESDAY
- THURSDAY
- FRIDAY
- SATURDAY
- SUNDAY

GRAND TOTALS ➡

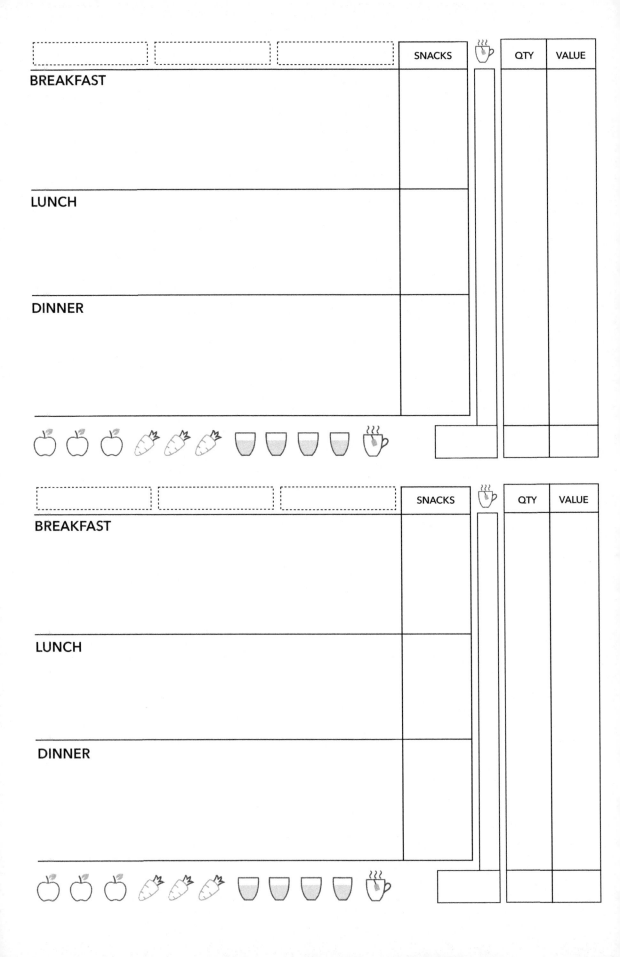

			SNACKS		QTY	VALUE

BREAKFAST

LUNCH

DINNER

			SNACKS		QTY	VALUE

BREAKFAST

LUNCH

DINNER

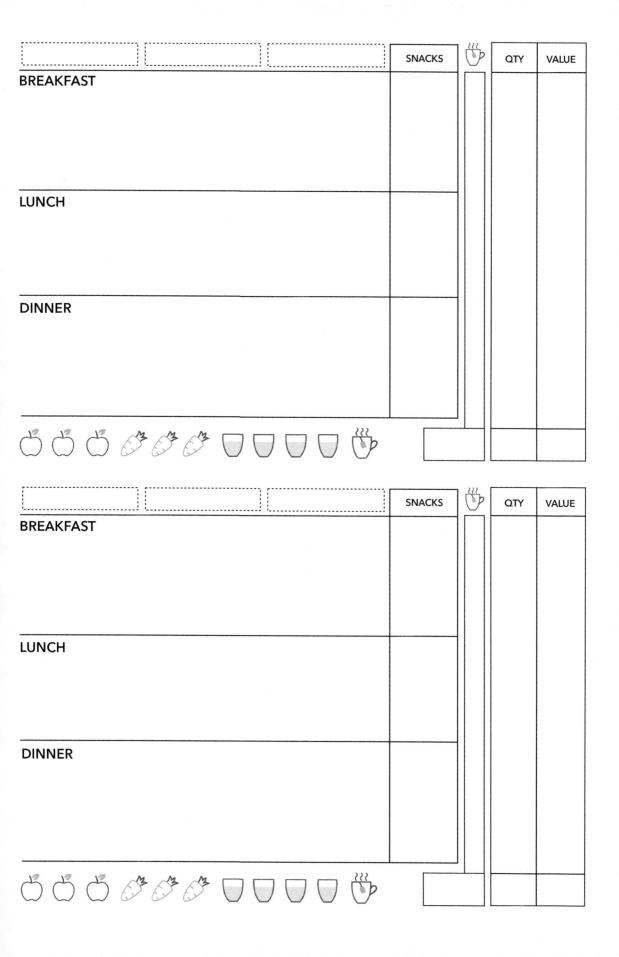

			SNACKS		QTY	VALUE

BREAKFAST

LUNCH

DINNER

			SNACKS		QTY	VALUE

BREAKFAST

LUNCH

DINNER

			SNACKS	☕	QTY	VALUE

BREAKFAST

LUNCH

DINNER

🍎 🍎 🍎 🥕 🥕 🥕 ☕ ☕ ☕ ☕ ☕

			SNACKS	☕	QTY	VALUE

BREAKFAST

LUNCH

DINNER

🍎 🍎 🍎 🥕 🥕 🥕 ☕ ☕ ☕ ☕ ☕

			SNACKS		QTY	VALUE
BREAKFAST						
LUNCH						
DINNER						

WEEK 9 - SEVEN DAY SUMMARY

		VALUE TOTALS	BEVERAGE TOTALS

Fruit - Veg - Water

- MONDAY
- TUESDAY
- WEDNESDAY
- THURSDAY
- FRIDAY
- SATURDAY
- SUNDAY

GRAND TOTALS

			SNACKS		QTY	VALUE

BREAKFAST

LUNCH

DINNER

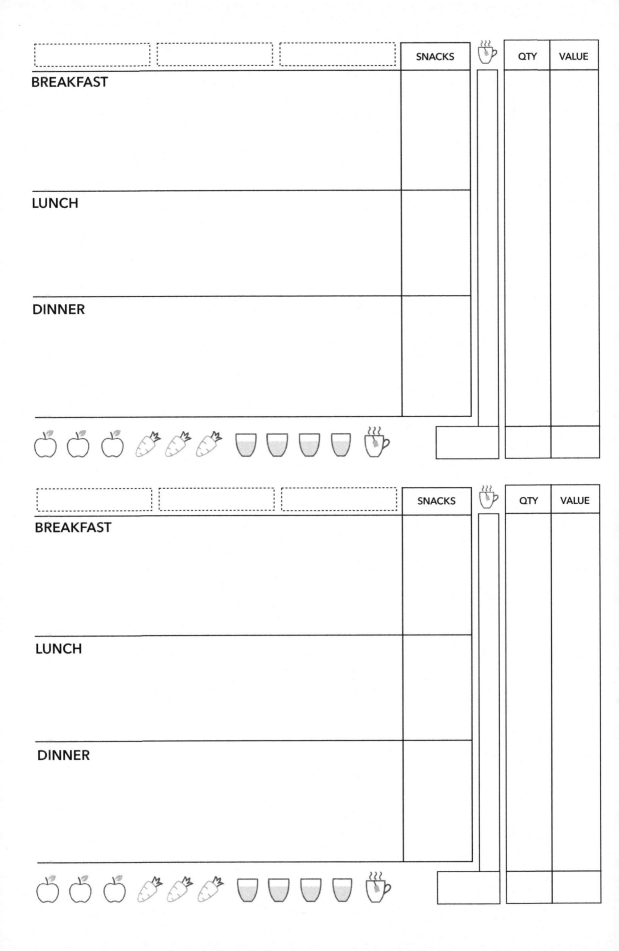

			SNACKS		QTY	VALUE

BREAKFAST

LUNCH

DINNER

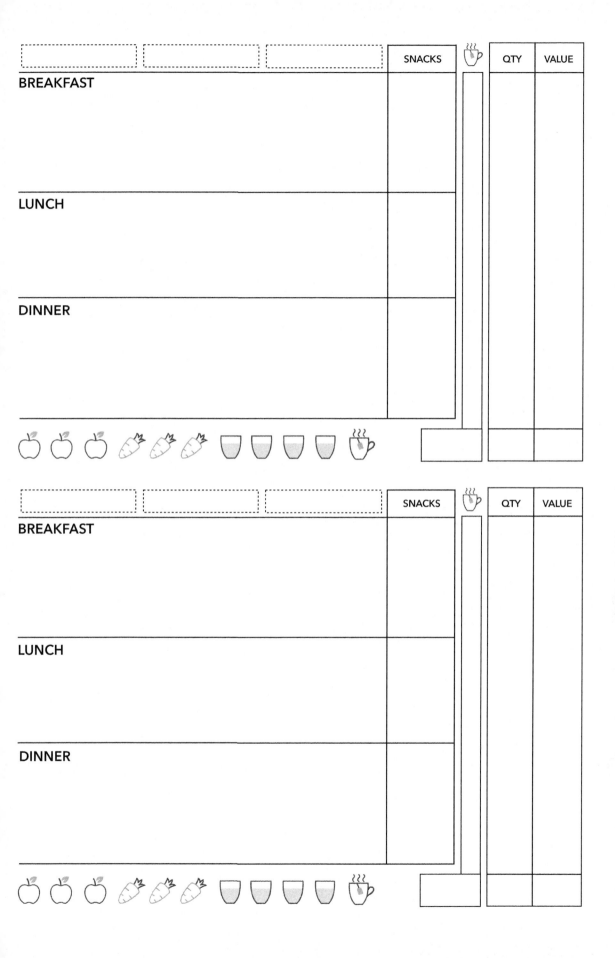

			SNACKS		QTY	VALUE

BREAKFAST

LUNCH

DINNER

			SNACKS		QTY	VALUE

BREAKFAST

LUNCH

DINNER

			SNACKS		QTY	VALUE
BREAKFAST						
LUNCH						
DINNER						

			SNACKS		QTY	VALUE
BREAKFAST						
LUNCH						
DINNER						

			SNACKS	☕	QTY	VALUE
BREAKFAST						
LUNCH						
DINNER						

🍎 🍎 🍎 🥕 🥕 🥕 🥛 🥛 🥛 🥛 ☕

WEEK 10 - SEVEN DAY SUMMARY

		VALUE TOTALS	BEVERAGE TOTALS

Fruit - Veg - Water

- MONDAY
- TUESDAY
- WEDNESDAY
- THURSDAY
- FRIDAY
- SATURDAY
- SUNDAY

GRAND TOTALS ➡

			SNACKS	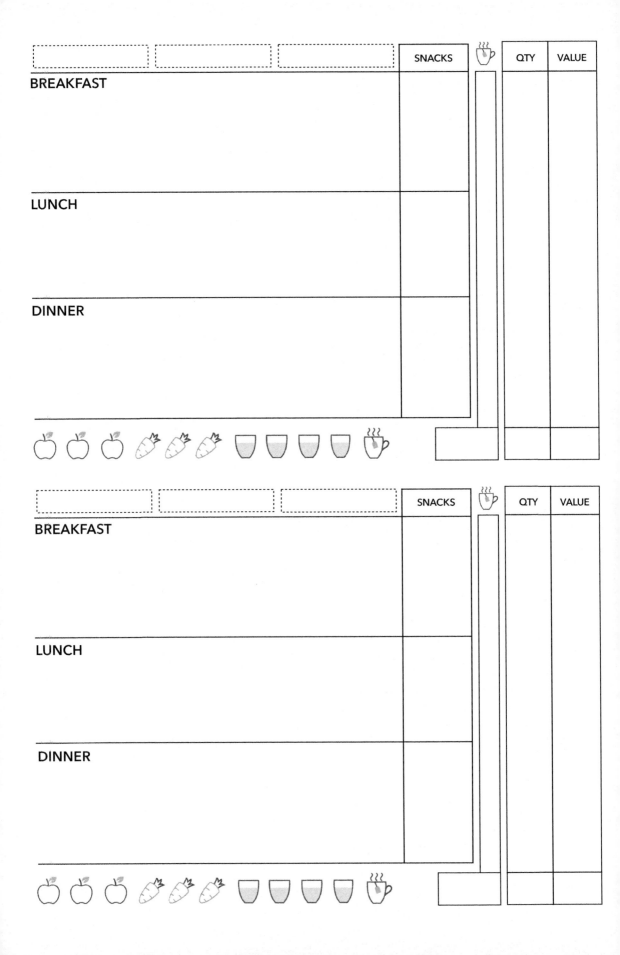	QTY	VALUE
BREAKFAST						
LUNCH						
DINNER						

			SNACKS		QTY	VALUE
BREAKFAST						
LUNCH						
DINNER						

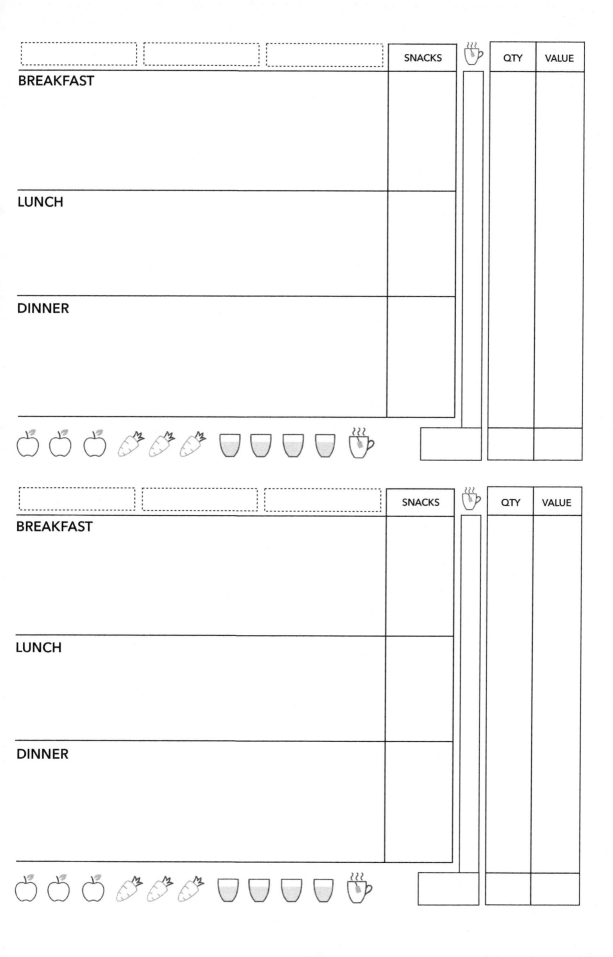

			SNACKS		QTY	VALUE

BREAKFAST

LUNCH

DINNER

			SNACKS		QTY	VALUE

BREAKFAST

LUNCH

DINNER

			SNACKS	☕	QTY	VALUE

BREAKFAST

LUNCH

DINNER

🍎 🍎 🍎 🥕 🥕 🥕 ☕ ☕ ☕ ☕ ☕

			SNACKS	☕	QTY	VALUE

BREAKFAST

LUNCH

DINNER

🍎 🍎 🍎 🥕 🥕 🥕 ☕ ☕ ☕ ☕ ☕

			SNACKS	☕	QTY	VALUE

BREAKFAST

LUNCH

DINNER

🍎 🍎 🍎 🥕 🥕 🥕 ⊔ ⊔ ⊔ ⊔ ☕

WEEK 11 - SEVEN DAY SUMMARY

	VALUE TOTALS	BEVERAGE TOTALS

Fruit - Veg - Water

- MONDAY
- TUESDAY
- WEDNESDAY
- THURSDAY
- FRIDAY
- SATURDAY
- SUNDAY

GRAND TOTALS ▶ ____ ____ ____   ▶ ____   ▶ ____

			SNACKS		QTY	VALUE
BREAKFAST						
LUNCH						
DINNER						

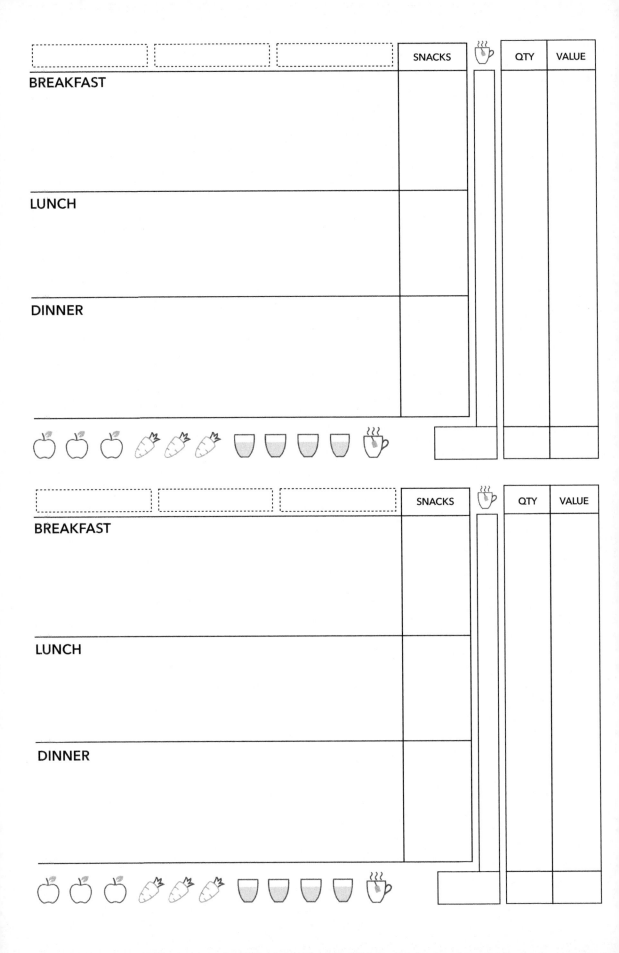

			SNACKS		QTY	VALUE
BREAKFAST						
LUNCH						
DINNER						

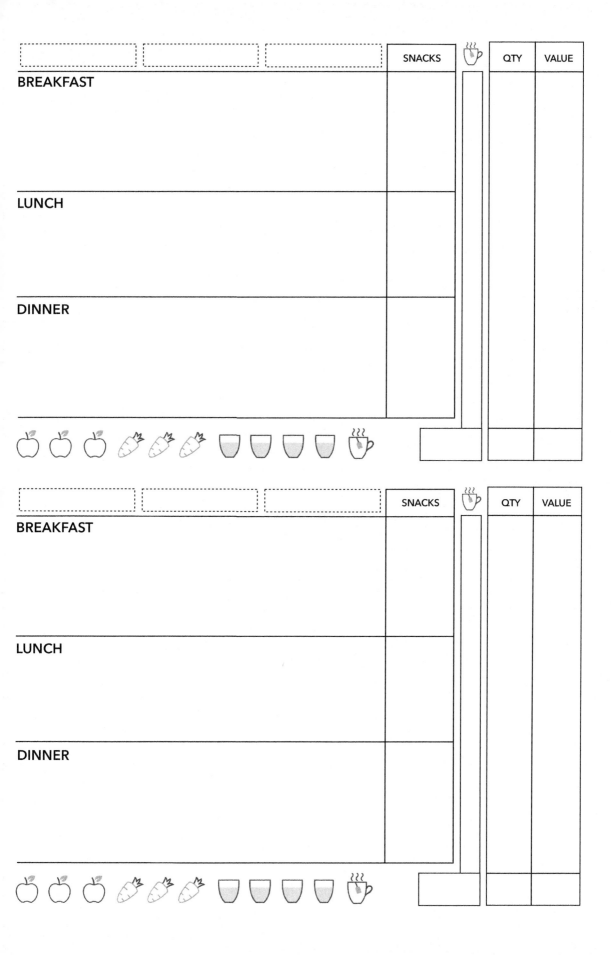

			SNACKS		QTY	VALUE

BREAKFAST

LUNCH

DINNER

			SNACKS		QTY	VALUE

BREAKFAST

LUNCH

DINNER

			SNACKS		QTY	VALUE
BREAKFAST						
LUNCH						
DINNER						

			SNACKS		QTY	VALUE
BREAKFAST						
LUNCH						
DINNER						

			SNACKS	☕	QTY	VALUE
BREAKFAST						
LUNCH						
DINNER						

🍎 🍎 🍎 🥕 🥕 🥕 🥛 🥛 🥛 🥛 ☕

WEEK 12 - SEVEN DAY SUMMARY

		VALUE TOTALS	BEVERAGE TOTALS

Fruit - Veg - Water

- MONDAY
- TUESDAY
- WEDNESDAY
- THURSDAY
- FRIDAY
- SATURDAY
- SUNDAY

GRAND TOTALS

ACTIVITY TRACKER - 10,000 STEPS...!

So where does the magic number come from? It's believed that the concept of 10,000 steps originated in Japan in the run-up to the 1964 Tokyo Olympics, says Catrine Tudor-Locke, an associate professor at the Pennington Biomedical Research Centre at Louisiana State University.

Pedometers became all the rage in the country as Olympic fever swept through Japanese society. One company came out with a device called a manpo-kei, which means 10,000 step meter.

Since then 10,000 steps has become a commonly-acknowledged goal for daily fitness across the world. The 10,000-step goal could be just right for you – and the benefits of a 30-minute extra walk to help hit your target helps:

- Lowers blood pressure
- Lowers depression
- Improves Sleep
- And makes you Super Fit

Set your goal and build up to the 10,000 steps per day.

Our activity tracker is set up so it acts like a graph allowing you to see your daily step totals at a glance.

Steps Range - 6,000 to 12,000 Steps - The Grey Box / Line is the Goal

For more information and to see a Graph Example: www.myfooddiary.co.uk
Select **>More** and then see **Activity Tracker**

| | MON | TUE | WED | THUR | FRI | SAT | SUN | **ACTIVITY NOTES** |

| 12 |
| 500 |
| 11 |
| 500 |
| 10 |
| 500 |
| 9 |
| 500 |
| 8 |
| 500 |
| 7 |
| 500 |
| 6 |

ACTIVITY NOTES

	MON	TUE	WED	THUR	FRI	SAT	SUN

12
500
11
500
10
500
9
500
8
500
7
500
6

12
500
11
500
10
500
9
500
8
500
7
500
6

12
500
11
500
10
500
9
500
8
500
7
500
6

12
500
11
500
10
500
9
500
8
500
7
500
6

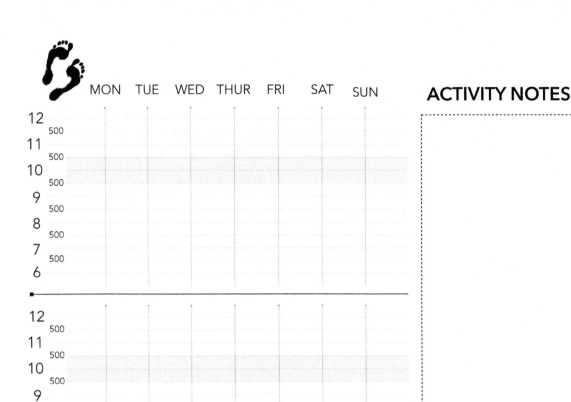

	MON	TUE	WED	THUR	FRI	SAT	SUN

ACTIVITY NOTES

12
500
11
500
10
500
9
500
8
500
7
500
6

12
500
11
500
10
500
9
500
8
500
7
500
6

12
500
11
500
10
500
9
500
8
500
7
500
6

12
500
11
500
10
500
9
500
8
500
7
500
6

ACTIVITY NOTES

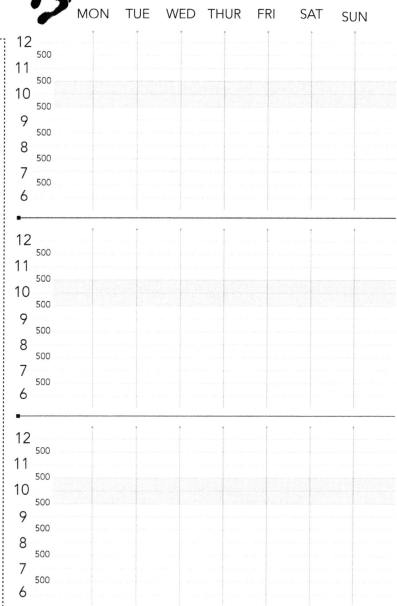

	MON	TUE	WED	THUR	FRI	SAT	SUN
12							
500							
11							
500							
10							
500							
9							
500							
8							
500							
7							
500							
6							

EXERCISE & FITNESS

9 MINUTES is all you need per day to help speed up your weight loss and increase your fitness and stamina levels. We have created a simple but effective workout routine for you. Simply choose the exercises that are right for you and when you feel to need to do more, select a harder more intense exercise.

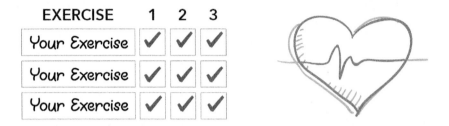

When you have completed your entire workout, give yourself a tick for each exercise performed. This gives a visual motivational calendar view of your weekly success - **You will be totally motivated to see your success!**

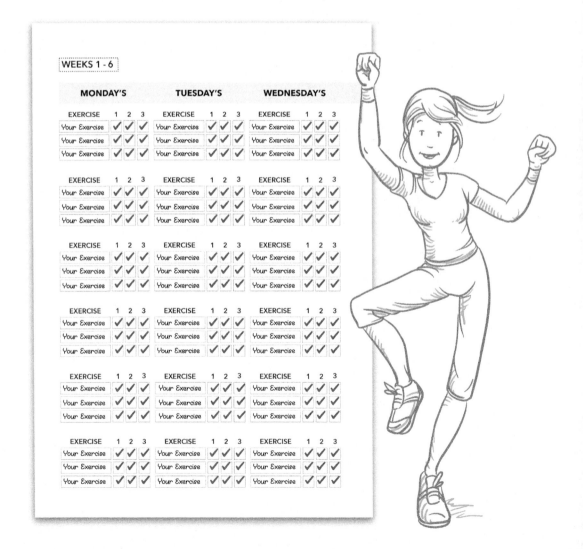

THE EXERCISES

Choose three exercises from the list below. Stick with your chosen exercises for the entire week and perform the following routine formula. When you feel ready, up your exercise to a more intensive one. * Feel Free to choose or make up your own exercises if you prefer.

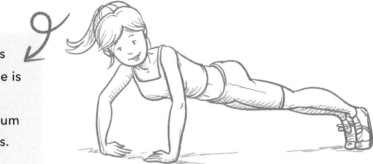

Try all the exercises once to see which one is right for you.
Follow the low, medium and high guidelines.

LOW Intensity Level	**MEDIUM** Intensity Level	**HIGH** Intensity Level
• Chair Squats	• Air Punches	• Jumping Jacks
• The Bridge	• Free Squats	• Burpees
• Quater Squats	• Lunges	• Mountain Climb
• The Plank	• Stair Walking	• Walking Lunges

THE EXERCISE FORMULA

Exercise **1** - 3 x 1 Minute Sets / 30 - 45 Seconds Rest.

(60 Seconds rest before next exercise)

Exercise **2** - 3 x 1 Minute Sets / 30 - 45 Seconds Rest.

(60 Seconds rest before next exercise)

Exercise **3** - 3 x 1 Minute Sets / 30 - 45 Seconds Rest.

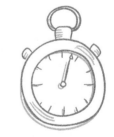

(Total Workout time with rest - Averages about 14 Minutes)

* You can increase your intensity by reducing your resting times, thus reducing your total workout time.

MONDAY'S				TUESDAY'S				WEDNESDAY'S			
EXERCISE	1	2	3	EXERCISE	1	2	3	EXERCISE	1	2	3

EXERCISE	1	2	3	EXERCISE	1	2	3	EXERCISE	1	2	3

EXERCISE	1	2	3	EXERCISE	1	2	3	EXERCISE	1	2	3

EXERCISE	1	2	3	EXERCISE	1	2	3	EXERCISE	1	2	3

EXERCISE	1	2	3	EXERCISE	1	2	3	EXERCISE	1	2	3

EXERCISE	1	2	3	EXERCISE	1	2	3	EXERCISE	1	2	3

THURSDAY'S				FRIDAY'S				SATURDAY'S			
EXERCISE	1	2	3	EXERCISE	1	2	3	EXERCISE	1	2	3
EXERCISE	1	2	3	EXERCISE	1	2	3	EXERCISE	1	2	3
EXERCISE	1	2	3	EXERCISE	1	2	3	EXERCISE	1	2	3
EXERCISE	1	2	3	EXERCISE	1	2	3	EXERCISE	1	2	3
EXERCISE	1	2	3	EXERCISE	1	2	3	EXERCISE	1	2	3
EXERCISE	1	2	3	EXERCISE	1	2	3	EXERCISE	1	2	3

WEEKS 7 - 12

MONDAY'S				TUESDAY'S				WEDNESDAY'S			

EXERCISE	1	2	3	EXERCISE	1	2	3	EXERCISE	1	2	3

EXERCISE	1	2	3	EXERCISE	1	2	3	EXERCISE	1	2	3

EXERCISE	1	2	3	EXERCISE	1	2	3	EXERCISE	1	2	3

EXERCISE	1	2	3	EXERCISE	1	2	3	EXERCISE	1	2	3

EXERCISE	1	2	3	EXERCISE	1	2	3	EXERCISE	1	2	3

EXERCISE	1	2	3	EXERCISE	1	2	3	EXERCISE	1	2	3

THURSDAY'S					FRIDAY'S					SATURDAY'S			
EXERCISE	1	2	3		EXERCISE	1	2	3		EXERCISE	1	2	3
EXERCISE	1	2	3		EXERCISE	1	2	3		EXERCISE	1	2	3
EXERCISE	1	2	3		EXERCISE	1	2	3		EXERCISE	1	2	3
EXERCISE	1	2	3		EXERCISE	1	2	3		EXERCISE	1	2	3
EXERCISE	1	2	3		EXERCISE	1	2	3		EXERCISE	1	2	3
EXERCISE	1	2	3		EXERCISE	1	2	3		EXERCISE	1	2	3

SLEEP TRACKER

While sleep requirements vary slightly from person to person, most healthy adults need between 7 to 9 hours of sleep per night to function at their best.

Sleep makes you feel better and does more than just make you feel refreshed.

A good regular sleeping patten helps you:

- Improve memory
- Improve creativity
- Improve attention
- Maintain a healthy weight
- Lowers stress levels
- Stops you feeling depressed
- and helps you live longer…!

A sleep tracker will help track the amount of hours you are getting. You want to aim for the same amount each night within 30 to 45 Minutes sleep range. But listen to your body - If you need the sleep, make sure you get it…!

Our sleep tracker is set up so it acts like a graph allowing you to see your sleep patten at a glance.

Example:

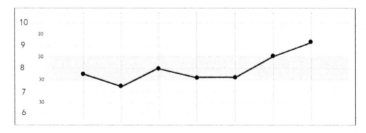

 MON   TUE   WED   THUR   FRI   SAT   SUN

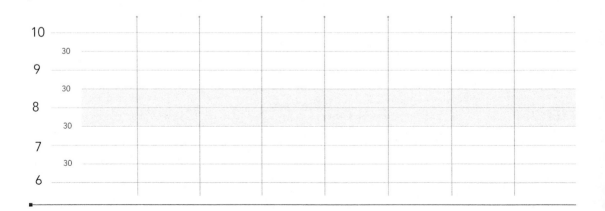

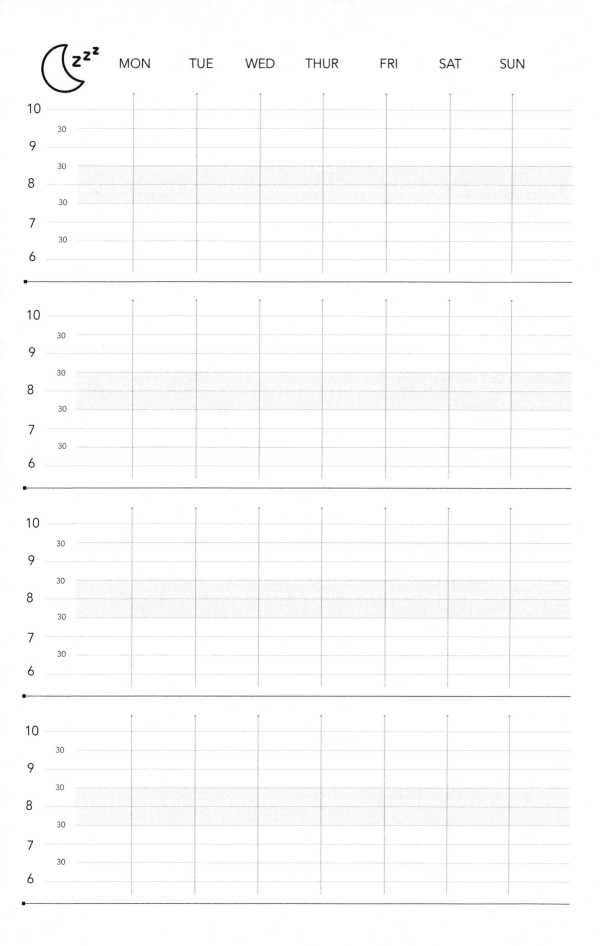

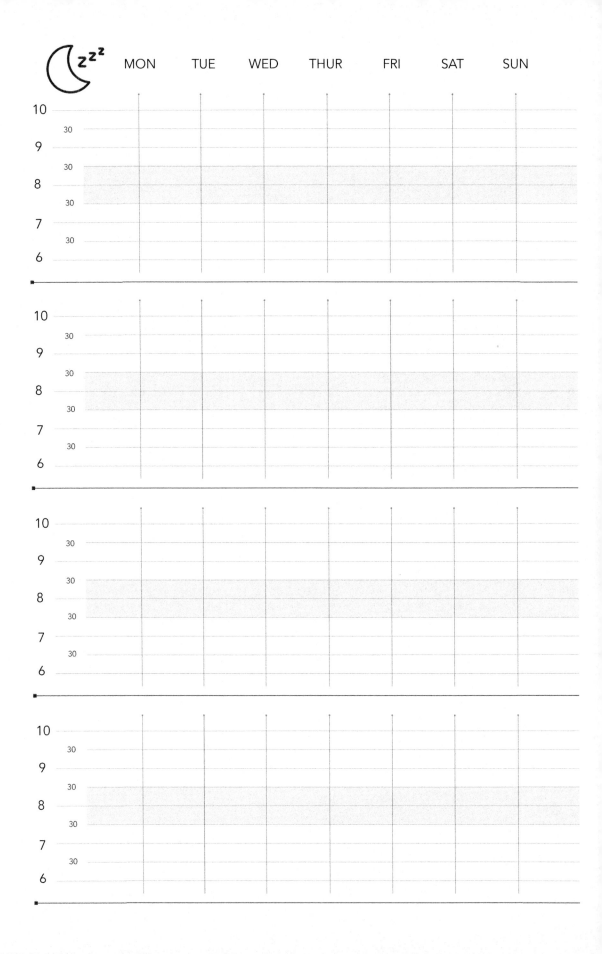

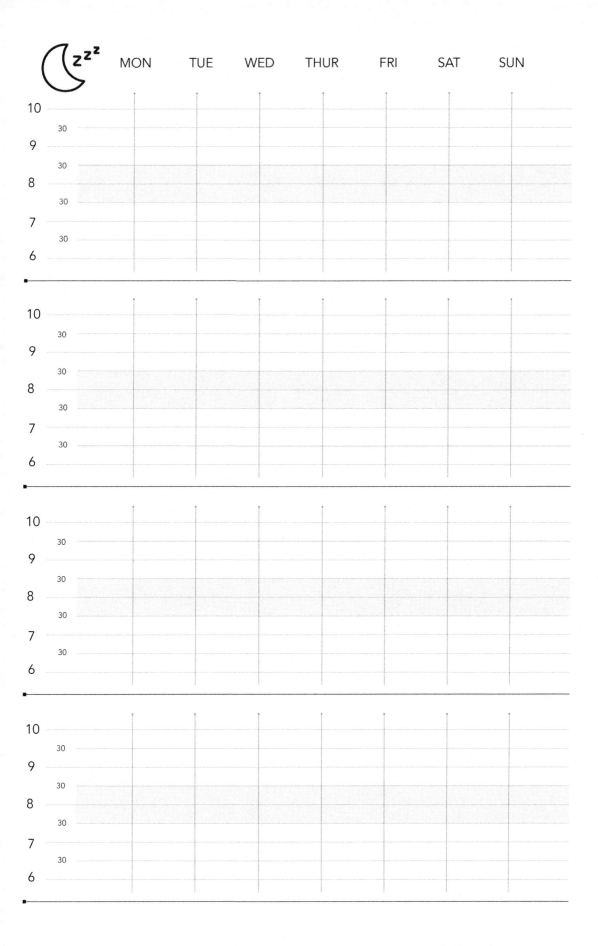